Copyright ©

Table of Contents

Braised Brisket with Dried Fruit

Roasted Salmon with Spicy Cranberry Relish

Quick Kale Dolmas

Chickpea Dumplings in Curried Tomato Sauce

Introduction

Many women are looking for that perfect pregnancy diet. One that will help them feel great, nourish their growing baby within, and perhaps help them not gain too much weight (pregnant women are like powerlifters after all).

But there is so much conflicting information out there.

- Eat mostly plants.
- Eat lots of protein.
- Don't eat salt.
- Do eat salt.
- Eat fish.
- Fish is too high in contaminants.

And then there are women who don't have the luxury of thinking about the perfect pregnancy diet as they are in the throws of Hyperemesis Gravidarum, a debilitating form of nausea and vomiting.

In this book, we'll cover some of the most common ideas around pregnancy diet and determine what's best for YOU.

Although pregnant women do not have to "eat for two", a healthy, balanced and varied diet that is rich in vitamins and minerals is important for both a mother and her baby. The mother's diet must provide sufficient energy (calories) and nutrients to meet her usual requirements, as well as the needs of the growing fetus, and enable the mother to lay down stores of nutrients required for the baby's development and for breastfeeding.

Pregnant women, as well as those planning for pregnancy, should follow a healthy, balanced diet. This can be achieved by following the usual guidelines, which are based around the five main food groups:

Bread, other cereals and potatoes. Foods in this group include breakfast cereals, pasta and rice. These foods should make up the main part of the diet. They are good sources of carbohydrate, protein and B vitamins, low in fat and filling. Whole-grain varieties contain more vitamins and minerals and breakfast cereals that contain added iron and folic acid are a good choice during pregnancy.

Meat, fish and alternatives. Alternatives include eggs, nuts, pulses (such as beans, lentils, chickpeas) and textured vegetable protein. These should be consumed in moderate amounts and lower fat versions selected whenever possible. They are a major source of protein, vitamins and minerals. Atleast one portion of oily fish (e.g. sardines or salmon) a week will ensure an adequate supply of omega-3 fatty acids.

Milk and dairy foods. These should be consumed in moderate amounts and lower fat versions are preferable. These foods are particularly high in calcium and good sources of protein. Skimmed and semi-skimmed milk contain just as much calcium and protein as whole milk. Foods containing fat and sugar. These foods add palat-ability to the diet but should be eaten infrequently.

Key pregnancy nutrition

A pregnant woman needs more calcium, folic acid, iron and protein than a woman who is not expecting, according to the American College of Obstetricians and Gynecologists (ACOG). Here is why these four nutrients are important.

Folic acid

Also known as folate when the nutrient is found in foods, folic acid is a B vitamin that is crucial in helping to prevent birth defects in the baby's brain and spinal cord, known as neural tube defects.

It may be hard to get the recommended amount of folic acid from diet alone. For that reason the March of Dimes, an organization dedicated to preventing birth defects, recommends that women who are trying to have a baby take a daily vitamin supplement containing 400 micrograms of folic acid per day for at least one month before becoming pregnant. During pregnancy, they advise women to increase the amount of folic acid to 600 micrograms a day, an amount commonly found in a daily prenatal vitamin. Food sources: leafy green vegetables, fortified or enriched cereals, breads and pastas, beans, citrus fruits.

Calcium:

This mineral is used to build a baby's bones and teeth. If a pregnant woman does not consume enough calcium, the mineral will be drawn from the mother's stores in her bones and given to the baby to meet the extra demands of pregnancy, according to the Academy of Nutrition and Dietetics. Many dairy products are also fortified with vitamin D, another nutrient that works with calcium to develop a baby's bones and teeth. Pregnant women age 19 and over need 1,000 milligrams of calcium a day; pregnant teens, ages 14 to 18, need 1,300 milligrams daily, according to ACOG. Food sources: milk, yogurt, cheese, calcium-fortified juices and foods, sardines or salmon with bones, some leafy greens (kale, bok choy).

Iron:

Pregnant women need 27 milligrams of iron a day, which is double the amount needed by women who are not expecting, according to ACOG. Additional amounts of the mineral are needed to make more blood to supply the baby with oxygen. Getting too little iron during pregnancy can lead to anemia, a condition resulting in fatigue and an increased risk of infections. To increase the absorption of iron, include a good source of vitamin C at the same meal when eating iron-rich foods, ACOG recommends. For example, have a glass of orange juice at breakfast with an iron-fortified cereal. Food sources: meat, poultry, fish, dried beans and peas, iron-fortified cereal.

Protein:

More protein is needed during pregnancy, but most women don't have problems getting enough protein-rich foods in their diets, said Sarah Krieger, a registered dietitian and spokeswoman on prenatal nutrition for the Academy of Nutrition and Dietetics in St. Petersburg, Florida. She described protein as "a builder nutrient," because it helps to build important organs for the baby, such as the brain and heart. Food sources: meat, poultry, fish, dried beans and peas, eggs, nuts, tofu.

Foods to eat

During pregnancy, the goal is to be eating nutritious foods most of the time, Krieger told Live Science. To maximize prenatal nutrition, she suggests emphasizing the following five food groups: fruits, vegetables, lean protein, whole grains and dairy products. When counseling pregnant women, Krieger recommends they fill half their plates with fruits and vegetables, a quarter of it with whole grains and a quarter of it with a source of lean protein, and to also have a dairy product at every meal.

Fruits and vegetables:

Pregnant women should focus on fruits and vegetables, particularly during the second and third trimesters, Krieger said. Get between five and 10 tennis ball-size servings of produce every day, she said. These colorful foods are low in calories and filled with fiber, vitamins and minerals.

Lean protein:

Pregnant women should include good protein sources at every meal to support the baby's growth, Krieger said. Protein-rich foods include meat, poultry, fish, eggs, beans, tofu, cheese, milk, nuts and seeds.

Whole grains:

These foods are an important source of energy in the diet, and they also provide fiber, iron and B-vitamins. At least half of a pregnant woman's carbohydrate choices each day should come from whole grains, such as oatmeal, whole-wheat pasta or breads and brown rice, Krieger said.

Dairy:

Aim for 3 to 4 servings of dairy foods a day, Krieger suggested. Dairy foods, such as milk, yogurt and cheese are good dietary sources of calcium, protein and vitamin D. In addition to a healthy diet, pregnant women also need to take a daily prenatal vitamin to obtain some of the nutrients that are hard to get from foods alone, such as folic acid and iron, according to ACOG. For women who take chewable prenatal vitamins, Krieger advised checking the product labels, because chewables might not have sufficient iron levels in them. Detailed information on healthy food choices and quantities to include at meals can also be found in the pregnancy section of the USDA's choosemyplate.gov.

Foods to limit

Caffeine:

Consuming fewer than 200 mg of caffeine a day, which is the amount found in one 12-ounce cup of coffee, is generally considered safe during pregnancy, according to a 2010 ACOG committee opinion, which was reaffirmed in 2013. The committee report said moderate caffeine consumption during pregnancy does not appear to contribute to miscarriage or premature birth.

Fish:

Fish is a good source of lean protein, and some fish, including salmon and sardines, also contain omega-3 fatty acids, a healthy fat that's good for the heart. It is safe for pregnant women to eat 8 to 12 ounces of cooked fish and seafood a week, according to ACOG. However, they should limit albacore or "white" tuna, which has high levels of mercury, to no more than 6 ounces a week, according to ACOG. Mercury is a metal that can be harmful to a baby's developing brain. Canned light tuna has less mercury than albacore "white" tuna and is safer to eat during pregnancy.

Foods to avoid

Alcohol:

Avoid alcohol during pregnancy, Krieger advised. Alcohol in the mother's blood can pass directly to the baby through the umbilical cord. Heavy use of alcohol during pregnancy has been linked with fetal alcohol spectrum disorders, a group of conditions that can include physical problems, as well as learning and behavioral difficulties in babies and children, according to the Centers for Disease Control and Prevention (CDC).

Fish with high levels of mercury:

Seafood such as swordfish, shark, king mackerel, marlin, orange roughy and tilefish are high in levels of methyl mercury, according to the Academy of Nutrition and Dietetics, and should be avoided during pregnancy. Methyl mercury is a toxic chemical that can pass through the placenta and can be harmful to an unborn baby's developing brain, kidneys and nervous system.

Unpasteurized food:

According to the USDA, pregnant women are at high risk for getting sick from two different types of food poisoning: listeriosis, caused by the Listeria bacteria, and toxoplasmosis, an infection caused by a parasite. The CDC says that Listeria infection may cause miscarriage, stillbirth, preterm labor, and illness or death in newborns. To avoid listeriosis, the USDA recommends avoiding the following foods during pregnancy:

Unpasteurized (raw) milk and foods made from it, such as feta, Brie, Camembert, blue-veined cheeses, queso blanco and queso fresco. Pasteurization involves heating a product to a high temperature to kill harmful bacteria.

Hot dogs, luncheon meats and cold cuts unless heated to steaming hot before eating to kill any bacteria.

Store-bought deli salads, such as ham salad, chicken salad, tuna salad and seafood salad.

Unpasteurized refrigerated meat spreads or pates.

Raw meat:

A mother can pass a Toxoplasma infection on to her baby, which can cause problems such as blindness and mental disability later in life, reports the CDC. To prevent toxoplasmosis, the USDA recommends avoiding the following foods during pregnancy:

Rare, raw or undercooked meats and poultry.

Raw fish, such as sushi, sashimi, ceviches and carpaccio.

Raw and undercooked shellfish, such as clams, mussels, oysters and scallops.

Some foods may increase a pregnant woman's risk for other types of food poisoning, including illness caused by salmonella and E. coli bacteria. Foodsafety.gov lists these foods to avoid during pregnancy, and why they pose a threat:

Raw or undercooked eggs, such as soft-cooked, runny or poached eggs.

Foods containing undercooked eggs, such as raw cookie dough or cake batter, tiramisu, chocolate mousse, homemade ice cream, homemade eggnog, Hollandaise sauce.

Raw or undercooked sprouts, such as alfalfa, clover.

Unpasteurized juice or cider.

Pregnancy diet misconceptions

Morning sickness:

When a mother-to-be is experiencing morning sickness, the biggest mistake she can make is thinking that if she doesn't eat, she'll feel better, Krieger said.

The exact causes of morning sickness are not known, but it may be caused by hormonal changes or lower blood sugar, according to the Mayo Clinic. This common complaint can bring on waves of nausea and vomiting in some women, especially during the first three months of pregnancy.

And "it's definitely not happening only in the morning," Krieger said. "It's any time of day." To ease morning sickness, it's better to eat small amounts of foods that don't have an odor, since smells can also upset the stomach, she suggested.

Food cravings

It is common for women to develop a sudden urge or a strong dislike for a food during pregnancy. Some common cravings are for sweets, salty foods, red meat or fluids, Krieger said. Often, a craving is a body's way of saying it needs a specific nutrient, such as more protein or additional liquids to quench a thirst, rather than a particular food, she said.

Eating for two:

When people say that a pregnant woman is "eating for two," it doesn't mean she needs to consume twice as much food or double her calories. "A woman is not eating for two during her first trimester," Krieger said. During the first three months, Krieger tells women that their calorie needs are basically the same as they were before pregnancy. During the first trimester, the recommended weight gain is between 1 and 4 pounds over the three-month period.

Krieger typically advises pregnant women to add 200 calories to their usual dietary intake during the second trimester, and to add 300 calories during their third trimester when the baby is growing quickly.

Weight gain during pregnancy

"Weight gain during pregnancy often has an ebb and a flow over the nine months," Krieger said. It's hard to measure where pregnancy weight is going, she said, adding that a scale does not reveal whether the pounds are going to a woman's body fat, baby weight or fluid gains.

When it comes to pregnancy weight gain, Krieger advises mothers-to-be to look at the big picture:

During regular prenatal checkups, focus on the fact that the baby is growing normally rather than worrying about the number on a scale.

The total number of calories that are needed per day during pregnancy depends on a woman's height, her weight before becoming pregnant, and how active she is on a daily basis. In general, underweight women need more calories during pregnancy; overweight and obese women need fewer of them. The Institute of Medicine (IOM) guidelines for total weight gain during a full-term pregnancy recommend that:

Underweight women, who have a Body Mass Index (BMI) below 18.5, should gain 28 to 40 lbs. (12.7 to 18 kilograms).

Normal weight women, who have a BMI of 18.5 to 24.9, should gain 25 to 35 lbs. (11.3 to 15.8 kg).

Overweight women, who have a BMI of 25.0 to 29.9, should gain 15 to 25 lbs. (6.8 to 11.3 kg).

Obese women, who have a BMI of 30.0 and above, should gain 11 to 20 lbs. (5 to 9 kg).

Rate of weight gain

The IOM guidelines suggest that pregnant women gain between 1 and 4.5 lbs. (0.45 to 2 kg) total during their first trimester of pregnancy. The guidelines recommend that underweight and normal-weight women gain, on average, about 1 pound every week during their second and third trimesters of pregnancy, and that overweight and obese women gain about half a pound every week in their second and third trimesters of pregnancy.

Twins

The IOM guidelines for pregnancy weight gain when a woman is having twins are as follows:

Underweight: 50 to 62 lbs. (22.6 kg to 28.1 kg).

Normal weight: 37 to 54 lbs. (16.7 to 24.5 kg).

Overweight: 31 to 50 lbs. (14 to 22.6 kg).

Obese: 25 to 42 lbs. (11.3 to 19 kg).

The effect of diet on gastrointestinal symptoms and morning sickness

Indigestion, heartburn and intestinal discomfort are common, especially in late pregnancy when the baby takes up more space and squashes internal organs. Women usually learn by experience which foods to avoid and this is unlikely to lead to any nutritional problems unless it involves foods that are a major source of important nutrients (e.g. all meat or dairy products). Eating small meals, avoiding fatty and spicy foods may help. Women who are experiencing constipation or haemorrhoids should increase the amount of fibre in the diet, by increasing intake of starchy carbohydrate foods, particularly whole-grain cereals and breads. An adequate fluid intake is also important, along with gentle exercise.

It is not unusual to have cravings for certain foods and aversions to other foods during pregnancy. The cause of these is also uncertain but may be due to altered taste perceptions. Dairy and sweet foods are most commonly reported as being craved and the most common aversions are to alcohol, caffeinated drinks and meats. As long as a healthy, varied diet is being consumed, there should not be cause for concern. Once the baby has been born, tastes usually return back to normal.

Food avoidance and risk of childhood food allergy

Infants whose parents have a history of allergic disease are more likely to develop allergies themselves and it has been suggested that by avoiding certain foods during pregnancy and breastfeeding mothers may help to prevent allergy in their infants. But there is little evidence to support this and others have suggested that exposure to these foods can actually help a baby develop tolerance to them. If there is strong family history of allergic disease (i.e. if either parent or a previous child has suffered from hayfever, asthma, eczema or other allergy), then it may be advisable to avoid peanuts or foods containing peanuts during pregnancy and while breastfeeding in order to reduce the risk of the infant developing a peanut allergy.

Dietary Guidelines for Pregnant Women

A woman who is pregnant or plans to get pregnant should start having proper nourishment right away. You can follow a 3-month pregnancy diet chart from the beginning, as it will help in building nutrition reserve that will supplement the growing baby right from conception. Eating healthy will provide you with essential nutrients that will strengthen your body and immune system, and enhance your metabolism. Before you follow a certain diet plan for pregnancy, it is recommended that you consult your gynaecologist.

Here are a few guidelines to follow when you are on a pregnancy diet:

Keep yourself hydrated through the day and drink as much water or juice as you can, at frequent intervals

Consume foods prepared with whole grains such as jowar,nachni, oats, barley recipes.

Consume fresh fruits and vegetables

Reduce the intake of sugar and sweet dishes to avoid chances of getting gestational diabetes

Avoid drinking alcohol and packaged juices, and steer clear of fried foods.

Apart from eating healthy, take the necessary supplements for iron, calcium, folic acid and vitamins, as suggested by your doctor. These help to avoid the possibility of neural tube defects affecting the baby and assist in the development of the brain and other organs

Essential fats like Omega 3 fats are essential for the body. SOurces of them are fish oils, walnuts, flax seeds

Early Morning

Morning sickness is part and parcel of pregnancy. Foods like lemon water with ginger, coconut water, or foods like dry biscuits help relieve morning sickness. Salads and curd help ease constipation and heartburn.

Breakfast

Breakfast is the most essential meal of the day, and it is mandatory for expecting women. Skipping breakfast can make you feel tired and lethargic. This is because you have been hungry during the night and that causes your blood sugar level to drop. You can start your day with nutritious breakfast as indicated below:

1 bowl of oatmeal, fresh fruits nuts, and a glass of milk – These have important vitamins and fibre.

1 plate rava upma or poha or vermicelli with eggs or vegetables such as sprouts – These nourish you with multi nutrients and fibre.-

2 chapatis and an omelette.-

A vegetable omelette or vegetable sandwich with cheese – the best source of proteins

2 parathas with fillings of dal, potatoes, carrots, spinach or mixed veggies with curd – these provide fibre, calcium and vitamins.

Lunch

Make the most of your lunchtime, and eat a balanced meal. You can choose from an array of dishes using pulses, dals, cereals, whole grains, nuts and fresh vegetables. These will provide you with the right amount of vitamins, fibre, and minerals. Use only healthy oils like rice bran oil, coconut oil, ghee, or olive oil for cooking. You may have salads or a bowl of soup made of vegetables as a pre-lunch snack. If you eat non-vegetarian food, you could include chicken and fish as they will provide a good amount of proteins, omega-3 and healthy fats. They also help in forming red blood cells.

Here are a few meal ideas:

2 rotis with dal, a bowl of curd and chicken or vegetable curry like mix veg, kofta, paneer and other vegetables. –

Any rice dish like chicken/egg or jeera and pea rice, vegetable rice, khichdi or lemon rice with raita or plain curd rice.

1 bowl of chicken curry with vegetables, roti and rice.

1 bowl of palak paneer with roti or rice. Spinach is rich in folic acid and iron and is perfect for pregnant women. Vitamin C improves iron absorption, so add a dash of lemon to palak.

Snacks

It is common to have frequent hunger pangs when you are pregnant. You have a life growing within you and your body is working day and night. You will definitely require more energy and hence more food. So, you should make it a habit to eat small frequent meals rather than 3 big meals. Here are some snack ideas for the evening.

Have fresh fruits or a fruit smoothie.

Munch a handful of walnuts, almonds or dates.

Vegetable or spinach idlis are filling and healthy.

Multi-grain bread or khakhra or bhakri are tasty and nutritious.

Carrot or lauki halwa made with jaggery or less sugar can help satiate that sweet tooth.

Daliya or uttapam with vegetables is a complete mini-meal.

Roasted chana, peanuts and dates are high in fibre and are a suitable cure for constipation.

Dinner

It is recommended that you keep your dinner light and eat early. This healthy habit will aid in proper digestion of food and help you have a good night's sleep. For dinner, you can repeat the ideas from lunch. Some more ideas for your dinner include:

Roti with dal, any vegetable of your choice, salad, and curd.

Vegetable pulao or chicken rice with vegetable raita.

Vegetable, cheese, paneer, or egg paratha with buttermilk.

Jowar/ bajra roti with ghee, dal/ chicken curry/ vegetables, and raita – these grains are easy to digest.

Mixed dal khichdi with vegetable curry and bowl of curd.

Pick a diet that packs the best nutrients for you and your baby. Do make sure you consult your gynaecologist or nutritionist before following any specific diet so that you have a healthy pregnancy.

Pregenancy diet recipes

Spinach & Mushroom Quiche

This healthy vegetarian quiche recipe is as simple as it gets. It's a quiche without the fussy crust! It's filled with sweet wild mushrooms and savory Gruyère cheese. Enjoy it for breakfast or brunch, or serve it with a light salad for lunch.

Ingredients

2 tablespoons extra-virgin olive oil

8 ounces sliced fresh mixed wild mushrooms such as cremini, shiitake, button and/or oyster mushrooms

1 ½ cups thinly sliced sweet onion

1 tablespoon thinly sliced garlic

5 ounces fresh baby spinach (about 8 cups), coarsely chopped

6 large eggs

¼ cup whole milk

¼ cup half-and-half

1 tablespoon Dijon mustard

1 tablespoon fresh thyme leaves, plus more for garnish

¼ teaspoon salt

¼ teaspoon ground pepper

1 ½ cups shredded Gruyère cheese

Directions

Step 1

Preheat oven to 375 degrees F. Coat a 9-inch pie pan with cooking spray; set aside.

Step 2

Heat oil in a large nonstick skillet over medium-high heat; swirl to coat the pan. Add mushrooms; cook, stirring occasionally, until browned and tender, about 8 minutes. Add onion and garlic; cook, stirring often, until softened and tender, about 5 minutes. Add spinach; cook, tossing constantly, until wilted, 1 to 2 minutes. Remove from heat.

Step 3

Whisk eggs, milk, half-and-half, mustard, thyme, salt and pepper in a medium bowl. Fold in the mushroom mixture and cheese. Spoon into the prepared pie pan. Bake until set and golden brown, about 30 minutes. Let stand for 10 minutes; slice. Garnish with thyme and serve.

Nutrition Facts

Serving Size: 1 Slice

Per Serving:

277 calories; 20 g total fat; 8.2 g saturated fat; 220 mg cholesterol; 443 mg sodium. 289 mg potassium;

6.8 g carbohydrates; 1.5 g fiber; 3 g sugar; 17.1 g protein; 2127 IU vitamin a iu; 11 mg vitamin c; 39 mcg folate; 358 mg calcium; 2 mg iron; 42 mg magnesium;

Exchanges:

1 1/2 Fat, 1 High-Fat Protein, 1 Medium-Fat Protein, 1 Vegetable

Irish Beef Stew

If you're looking for a healthy beef stew recipe that delivers on comfort, look no further. This one-pot Irish beef stew is packed with veggies and rich meaty flavor. Make this Irish beef stew recipe with Guinness--a dark, malty Irish stout--to keep it authentic. Serve with a side of Irish soda bread to sop up the leftovers.

Ingredients

2 ¼ pounds boneless chuck roast, trimmed and cut into 1 1/2-inch pieces

¾ teaspoon salt

½ teaspoon ground pepper

2 tablespoons canola oil, divided

1 small yellow onion, chopped

3 medium carrots, diagonally sliced into 1-inch pieces

3 stalks celery, cut into 1-inch pieces

1 tablespoon tomato paste

1 (12 fluid ounce) bottle stout beer (such as Guinness)

2 teaspoons chopped fresh thyme

4 cups low-sodium beef broth

1 ½ pounds baby Yukon Gold potatoes, halved

2 tablespoons cornstarch

2 tablespoons cold water

2 tablespoons chopped fresh flat-leaf parsley, plus more for garnish

Directions

Step 1

Sprinkle beef all over with salt and pepper. Heat 1 tablespoon oil in a large heavy pot over medium-high heat. Add half of the beef; cook, turning to brown on 2 or 3 sides, about 3 minutes per side. Transfer the browned beef to a bowl; repeat the process with the remaining beef and 1 tablespoon oil.

Step 2

Add onion, carrots and celery to the drippings in the pot; cook, stirring often, until the vegetables begin to soften, about 4 minutes. Add tomato paste; cook, stirring constantly, for 1 minute. Add beer and thyme; cook, scraping the bottom of the pot to release any browned bits, until the liquid is slightly reduced, about 2 minutes. Add broth and the beef (with any accumulated juices in bowl); bring the mixture to a boil over medium-high heat. Reduce heat to medium-low; cover and cook until the beef is mostly tender, about 1 hour, 10 minutes. Stir in potatoes; cover and cook until the beef and potatoes are tender, 15 to 20 minutes.

Step 3

Whisk cornstarch and cold water in a small bowl. Increase heat to high; add the cornstarch mixture and cook, stirring constantly, until thickened, about 2 minutes. Remove from heat; stir in parsley. If desired, garnish with additional parsley.

Tips

To make ahead: Refrigerate in an airtight container for up to 3 days or freeze for up to 6 months. Thaw (if frozen) and reheat before serving.

Nutrition Facts

Serving Size: 2 1/4 Cups

Per Serving:

405 calories; 11.9 g total fat; 3.1 g saturated fat; 102 mg cholesterol; 704 mg sodium. 904 mg potassium; 32.1 g carbohydrates; 3.5 g fiber; 4 g sugar; 37.1 g protein; 5347 IU vitamin a iu; 14 mg vitamin c; 39 mcg folate; 49 mg calcium; 4 mg iron; 53 mg magnesium;

Exchanges:

4 1/2 Lean Protein, 1 1/2 Starch, 1 Fat, 1 Vegetable

Winter Greens Salad with Pomegranate & Kumquats

Kumquats deliver a piquant burst of citrus, especially when eaten skins, seeds and all. Here we toss them with a trio of greens for their vivid orange color as much as their zestiness. Pomegranate seeds and pistachios bring a jewel-like finish.

Ingredients

6 tablespoons pomegranate juice

½ teaspoon orange zest

1 ½ tablespoons orange juice

1 ½ teaspoons cornstarch

1 ½ teaspoons sugar

⅛ teaspoon garlic salt

¼ cup extra-virgin olive oil

2 heads Belgian endive, trimmed, leaves separated

1 small head radicchio, torn into small pieces

5 cups baby bitter greens, such as kale, arugula and/or frisée

1 cup pomegranate arils or raspberries

½ cup kumquats, thinly sliced, or orange segments

¼ cup toasted walnuts

¼ cup toasted pepitas or pistachios

Directions

Step 1

Combine pomegranate juice, orange zest, orange juice, cornstarch, sugar and garlic salt in a small saucepan and whisk well. Heat over medium-high heat, whisking constantly, until the mixture begins to boil, darkens and turns more translucent, about 5 minutes. Remove from heat and let cool to room temperature, about 20 minutes. Whisk in oil.

Step 2

Arrange endive, radicchio and baby greens on a platter. Top with pomegranate arils (or raspberries) and kumquats (or oranges) and drizzle with the dressing. Sprinkle with walnuts and pepitas (or pistachios).

Nutrition Facts

Serving Size: 2 1/2 Cups

Per Serving:

337 calories; 13 g total fat; 2.1 g saturated fat; 62 mg cholesterol; 644 mg sodium. 860 mg potassium; 27.9 g carbohydrates; 6.3 g fiber; 16 g sugar; 29.7 g protein; 5958 IU vitamin a iu; 80 mg vitamin c; 91 mcg folate; 194 mg calcium; 2 mg iron; 95 mg magnesium; 1 g added sugar;

Exchanges:

6 1/2 Fat, 3 Lean Protein, 2 Vegetable

Reuben Casserole

This Reuben casserole recipe has all the delicious elements of a Reuben sandwich with much less sodium and calories. Thinly sliced angel hair cabbage cooked with a splash of vinegar stands in for the sauerkraut, and lower-sodium deli turkey adds a rich, meaty flavor in place of the traditional corned beef.

Ingredients

3 tablespoons extra-virgin olive oil, divided

1 (10 ounce) package angel hair coleslaw mix or 5 cups very thinly sliced green cabbage

1 cup chopped yellow onion

⅛ teaspoon salt

2 tablespoons cider vinegar

1 ¼ cups shredded Swiss cheese

2 tablespoons chopped kosher dill pickle

⅓ pound sliced reduced-sodium deli turkey, coarsely chopped

⅓ cup mayonnaise

2 tablespoons no-salt-added ketchup

3 slices seeded rye bread, torn into pieces

Directions

Step 1

Preheat oven to 350 degrees F. Coat a 2-quart (7-by-11-inch) baking dish with cooking spray. Heat 1 tablespoon oil in a large nonstick skillet over medium-high heat. Add cabbage, onion and salt; cook, stirring often, until the cabbage wilts and the cabbage and onion begin to brown, about 5 minutes. Stir in vinegar and remove from heat. Transfer the mixture to the prepared baking dish.

Step 2

Sprinkle one-third of the cheese evenly over the cabbage mixture; sprinkle with pickle, then turkey, then another third of the cheese. Stir together mayonnaise and ketchup in a small bowl; spread over the top cheese layer. Sprinkle with the remaining cheese.

Step 3

Pulse bread in a food processor until coarse breadcrumbs form. Toss the breadcrumbs and the remaining 2 tablespoons oil in a small bowl; sprinkle over the top cheese layer.

Step 4

Bake the casserole until it's hot throughout, the cheese is melted and the breadcrumbs are light golden brown, about 20 minutes. Serve hot.

Nutrition Facts

Serving Size: 1 Cup

Per Serving:

338 calories; 23.9 g total fat; 6.7 g saturated fat; 7 mg cholesterol; 493 mg sodium. 243 mg potassium; 17 g carbohydrates; 3 g fiber; 6 g sugar; 14 g protein; 37 IU vitamin a iu; 25 mg vitamin c; 58 mcg folate; 246 mg calcium; 1 mg iron; 29 mg magnesium;

Exchanges:

3 Fat, 1 High-Fat Protein, 1 Lean Protein, 1 Vegetable, 1/2 Starch

Mini Cauliflower-Crust Pizzas

This gluten-free pizza recipe uses muffin tins to create perfectly portioned mini pizzas perfect for lunch or dinner. Cauliflower acts as the base of the crust while the classic toppings of bell pepper, black olives, pepperoni and ooey-gooey cheese promise to satisfy your strongest pizza cravings.

Ingredients

2 (10 ounce) packages cauliflower florets or 1 (2-pound) head cauliflower, cored and cut into florets

1 large egg, beaten

¼ cup almond flour

2 tablespoons grated Parmesan cheese

¼ teaspoon garlic powder

¼ teaspoon onion powder

3 ¼ cups shredded part-skim mozzarella cheese

½ cup pizza sauce

½ cup chopped red bell pepper

⅓ cup sliced ripe black olives

8 slices turkey pepperoni (about 1 ounce), quartered

Chopped fresh basil

Directions

Step 1

Position racks in upper and lower thirds of oven; preheat to 425 degrees F. Soak a paper towel with oil and use it to grease 2 nonstick muffin tins (you'll need 18 regular muffin cups). (Alternatively, line 2 stainless-steel muffin tins with 18 paper liners, and coat the liners with cooking spray.)

Step 2

Place cauliflower florets in a food processor and pulse until the cauliflower looks like rice, 4 to 5 pulses, stopping to scrape down the sides as needed. Transfer to a medium microwaveable glass bowl; microwave on High until tender, about 5 minutes. Let cool for 10 minutes. Place the cooled cauliflower in a clean towel; gather it to form a bundle and squeeze out as much moisture from the cauliflower as possible. Return the cauliflower to the bowl; add egg, almond flour, Parmesan, garlic powder, onion powder and 2 cups mozzarella. Stir with a fork until combined.

Step 3

Spoon the mixture evenly into the 18 prepared muffin cups (about 2 tablespoons per cup). Using your fingertips, press the mixture into the bottoms, making a slight indentation to shape the crusts. Bake until lightly browned, 18 to 20 minutes, rotating the pans between the racks halfway through baking.

Step 4

Remove the crusts from the oven; top each with about 1 1/2 teaspoons pizza sauce and sprinkle evenly with the remaining 1 1/4 cups mozzarella. Top evenly with bell pepper, olives and pepperoni. Continue baking until the pizzas are golden brown and the cheese has melted, 8 to 10 minutes.

Step 5

Let cool in the pans for 5 minutes. Remove the pizzas from the pans and transfer to a wire rack; let cool for 10 minutes. Remove paper liners, if necessary. Sprinkle with basil. Serve hot or at room temperature.

Tips

To make ahead: Refrigerate in an airtight container for up to 1 week. To reheat, wrap in foil and bake at 450 degrees F until hot, about 10 minutes.

Nutrition Facts

Serving Size: 3 Mini Pizzas

Per Serving:

259 calories; 15.2 g total fat; 7.9 g saturated fat; 77 mg cholesterol; 694 mg sodium. 537 mg potassium; 11.8 g carbohydrates; 2.8 g fiber; 4 g sugar; 20 g protein; 1130 IU vitamin a iu; 64 mg vitamin c; 83 mcg folate; 487 mg calcium; 1 mg iron; 41 mg magnesium;

Exchanges:

2 1/2 Medium-Fat Protein, 1 1/2 Vegetable, 1/2 Lean Protein

Baked Halibut with Brussels Sprouts & Quinoa

Fish plus two sides? It seems fancy but this healthy dinner comes together

Ingredients

1 pound Brussels sprouts, trimmed and sliced

1 fennel bulb, trimmed and cut into strips

1 tablespoon plus 1 teaspoon olive oil, divided

½ teaspoon salt, divided

½ teaspoon ground pepper, divided

1 (1 pound) halibut fillet, cut into 4 portions

4 cloves garlic, minced, divided

3 tablespoons lemon juice

2 tablespoons unsalted butter, melted

2 cups cooked quinoa (see Associated Recipes)

¼ cup chopped sun-dried tomatoes

¼ cup chopped pitted Kalamata olives

2 tablespoons chopped fresh Italian parsley or fennel
fronds

Directions

Step 1

Position racks in upper and lower thirds of oven;
preheat to 400 degrees F.

Step 2

Combine Brussels sprouts, fennel, 1 Tbsp. oil, and 1/4
tsp. each salt and pepper in a large bowl; toss to
coat. Spread in a single layer on a large rimmed
baking sheet. Bake, stirring occasionally, until tender,
20 to 25 minutes.

Step 3

Meanwhile, place halibut on another large rimmed baking sheet and top with half of the garlic and the remaining 1/4 tsp. each salt and pepper. Combine lemon juice and melted butter in a small bowl. Drizzle or brush half of the mixture over the fish. Bake until the fish is opaque and flakes easily with a fork, 12 to 15 minutes.

Step 4

Meanwhile, combine quinoa, the remaining 1 tsp. oil, sun-dried tomatoes, olives, and parsley (or fennel fronds) in a medium bowl.

Step 5

Add the remaining garlic to the lemon-butter mixture. Pour the mixture over the vegetables and bake for 1 minute more. Serve the halibut and vegetables alongside the quinoa mixture.

Nutrition Facts

Serving Size: 3 Oz. Fish + 1 Cup Vegetables + 1/2 Cup Quinoa

Per Serving:

406 calories; 17.1 g total fat; 5.3 g saturated fat; 71 mg cholesterol; 560 mg sodium. 1379 mg potassium; 36.1 g carbohydrates; 7.9 g fiber; 5 g sugar; 29.7 g protein; 1904 IU vitamin a iu; 97 mg vitamin c; 146 mcg folate; 108 mg calcium; 4 mg iron; 126 mg magnesium;

Lasagna Soup

This quick and healthy lasagna soup recipe has all the comforting flavors of classic lasagna with plenty of tomatoes, Italian turkey sausage and lasagna noodles broken into bite-size bits. A dollop of ricotta cheese mixed with mozzarella and Parmesan adds a creamy finishing touch. Serve the soup with a green salad and crusty bread to sop up what's left in the bowl for an easy healthy dinner that's ready in under 30 minutes.

Ingredients

2 tablespoons extra-virgin olive oil

1 cup chopped yellow onion

6 ounces hot Italian turkey sausage, casings removed

3 cloves garlic, finely chopped

1 tablespoon tomato paste

1 (28 ounce) can no-salt added crushed tomatoes

4 cups water

2 cups low-sodium chicken broth

1 tablespoon sugar

¼ teaspoon salt

6 ½ lasagna noodles (about 6 ounces), preferably whole-wheat, broken into 1 1/2-inch pieces

1 teaspoon balsamic vinegar

¾ cup part-skim ricotta cheese

½ cup shredded mozzarella cheese

2 tablespoons grated Parmesan cheese

2 tablespoons chopped fresh basil

Directions

Step 1

Heat oil in a large pot over medium-high heat. Add onion and cook, stirring occasionally, until almost translucent, about 5 minutes. Push onions to one side of the pot and add sausage to the other side. Cook, breaking up the sausage into small pieces with a wooden spoon, until browned, about 4 minutes. Add garlic and tomato paste; cook, stirring constantly, until the tomato paste is heated through, about 2 minutes. Add tomatoes, water, broth, sugar and salt; bring to a boil over high heat. Add lasagna noodles and stir to separate. Cook, stirring occasionally, until the pasta is just cooked through but not completely soft, 8 to 10 minutes. Remove from heat and stir in vinegar.

Step 2

Meanwhile, combine ricotta, mozzarella and Parmesan in a small bowl; set aside.

 Step 3

Ladle the soup into 6 bowls. Top each serving with a dollop of the ricotta mixture. Sprinkle with basil.

Nutrition Facts

Serving Size: 1 1/2 Cups

Per Serving:

351 calories; 13.9 g total fat; 4.7 g saturated fat; 34 mg cholesterol; 457 mg sodium. 684 mg potassium; 35.6 g carbohydrates; 6.8 g fiber; 9 g sugar; 19.9 g protein; 1386 IU vitamin a iu; 11 mg vitamin c; 13 mcg folate; 184 mg calcium; 4 mg iron; 15 mg magnesium; 2 g added sugar;

Exchanges:

2 Vegetable, 1 1/2 Starch, 1 Fat, 1 Medium-Fat Protein, 1/2 High-Fat Protein

Braised Brisket with Dried Fruit

This recipe features a brisket rub to rule all other brisket rubs. Covering the brisket with parchment paper before putting the lid on the pot is a classic French technique that creates a more richly flavored sauce.

Ingredients

3 whole star anise

4 teaspoons unsweetened cocoa powder

4 teaspoons ground sumac (see Tips)

2 teaspoons Urfa pepper (see Tips) or crushed red pepper

1 ¼ teaspoons ground cinnamon, preferably Vietnamese

4 pounds beef brisket, trimmed

½ teaspoon kosher salt

2 tablespoons extra-virgin olive oil

4 medium white onions, sliced

8 cloves garlic, minced

¼ cup dried apricots

¼ cup dried cranberries

¼ cup pitted prunes

¼ cup golden raisins

1 medium orange, cut into wedges

4 cups low-sodium beef broth

Directions

Step 1

Preheat oven to 325 degrees F.

Step 2

Finely grind star anise in a spice grinder or with a mortar and pestle. Transfer to a small bowl and stir in cocoa, sumac, pepper and cinnamon.

Step 3

Season brisket with salt and 2 tablespoons of the spice blend. Heat oil in a large ovenproof pot over high heat. Add the brisket and cook until browned, about 4 minutes per side. Transfer the brisket to a plate.

Step 4

Reduce heat to medium, add onions to the pot and cook, stirring often, until softened, about 10 minutes. Add garlic, apricots, cranberries, prunes, raisins, orange wedges and the remaining spice blend. Cook, stirring often, for 3 minutes more. Stir in broth and bring to a simmer. Return the brisket to the pot.

Step 5

Cover the brisket with a piece of parchment paper and put the lid on the pot. Transfer to the oven and bake until the brisket is fork-tender, about 3 1/2 hours.

Step 6

Transfer the brisket to a clean cutting board. Loosely cover with foil and let rest for 10 minutes. Slice the brisket against the grain and serve with the sauce.

Tips

Tips: Made from the tart red berries of the Mediterranean sumac bush, ground sumac has a fruity, sour flavor. Find this bright red spice in Middle Eastern markets, well-stocked supermarkets and online.

Urfa is a smoky, mildly hot Turkish chile pepper. Find the jars of dried flakes at specialty shops and online. Equipment: Spice grinder or mortar and pestle; parchment paper

Nutrition Facts

Serving Size: 3 Oz Cooked Meat, 1/2 Cup Sauce

Per Serving:

290 calories; 9.3 g total fat; 2.8 g saturated fat; 98 mg cholesterol; 320 mg sodium. 758 mg potassium;

15.7 g carbohydrates; 2.2 g fiber; 10 g sugar; 35.5 g protein; 279 IU vitamin a iu; 10 mg vitamin c; 31 mcg folate; 52 mg calcium; 4 mg iron; 48 mg magnesium; 2 g added sugar;

Roasted Salmon with Spicy Cranberry Relish

This ruby-red cranberry relish recipe gets refreshing crunch from apple and celery. It's also delightful alongside a roast chicken or pork loin.

Ingredients

2 ½ pounds skin-on salmon fillet

2 cloves garlic, peeled and chopped

1 ½ teaspoons kosher salt, divided

½ teaspoon whole black peppercorns, cracked

1 lemon, zested and cut into wedges

2 tablespoons extra-virgin olive oil, divided

2 teaspoons Dijon mustard

2 cups cranberries, fresh or frozen (8 ounces)

1 small shallot, minced

1 serrano pepper, seeded

1 medium Granny Smith apple, peeled and finely diced

1 stalk celery, finely diced

1 tablespoon balsamic vinegar

2 tablespoons chopped fresh parsley, divided

Directions

Step 1

Preheat oven to 400 degrees F. Line a rimmed baking sheet with parchment paper.

Step 2

Place salmon on the prepared pan. Mash garlic, 1 teaspoon salt, peppercorns and lemon zest into a paste with a fork or a mortar and pestle. Transfer to a small bowl and stir in 1 tablespoon oil and mustard. Spread on the salmon. Bake until the flesh flakes easily with a fork, 10 to 15 minutes.

Step 3

Meanwhile, pulse cranberries, shallot and serrano in a food processor until finely chopped. Transfer to a medium bowl and stir in apple, celery, vinegar, 1 tablespoon parsley and the remaining 1 tablespoon oil and 1/2 teaspoon salt.

Step 4

Sprinkle the salmon with the remaining 1 tablespoon parsley and serve with the relish and lemon wedges.

Tips

To make ahead: Refrigerate relish (Step 3) for up to 1 day.

Nutrition Facts

Serving Size: 4 Ounces Salmon And 1/3 Cup Relish

Per Serving:

229 calories; 8.8 g total fat; 1.8 g saturated fat; 66 mg cholesterol; 452 mg sodium. 603 mg potassium; 7.6 g carbohydrates; 1.7 g fiber; 4 g sugar; 28.6 g protein; 371 IU vitamin a iu; 10 mg vitamin c; 21 mcg folate; 65 mg calcium; 1 mg iron; 45 mg magnesium;

Quick Kale Dolmas

For a quick version of stuffed grape leaves, we've put all the flavors of a traditional dolma recipe into a cooked filling that's simply wrapped in blanched kale leaves--no need to simmer for hours.

Ingredients

16 medium kale leaves, stems trimmed, plus 4 cups chopped (from 2 large bunches)

½ cup low-fat plain Greek yogurt

1 teaspoon lemon zest

3 tablespoons lemon juice, divided

1 teaspoon salt, divided

½ teaspoon ground pepper, divided

1 tablespoon extra-virgin olive oil

1 medium onion, chopped

3 cloves garlic, minced

1 pound lean ground beef

2 cups cooked brown rice (see Tip)

½ cup chopped fresh parsley

2 tablespoons chopped fresh dill

Directions

Step 1

Bring a large pot of water to a boil. Add kale leaves and cook until bright green and very soft, 3 to 4 minutes. Using tongs, transfer the leaves to a clean kitchen towel and pat dry. Drain the water and wipe out the pot.

Step 2

Combine yogurt, 1 1/2 tablespoons lemon juice and 1/4 teaspoon each salt and pepper in a small bowl. Set aside.

Step 3

Heat oil, onion, garlic and chopped kale in the pot over medium-high heat. Cook, stirring occasionally and adding water 1 tablespoon at a time to prevent burning, until the vegetables are almost tender, about 5 minutes. Add beef and cook, breaking up with a wooden spoon, until browned, about 4 minutes. Stir in rice, parsley, dill, lemon zest and the remaining 1 1/2 tablespoons lemon juice, 3/4 teaspoon salt and 1/4 teaspoon pepper; cook, stirring, until hot, about 2 minutes. Remove from heat.

Step 4

Lay one of the kale leaves horizontally on a clean cutting board. Place a generous 1/4 cup of the beef mixture in the center. Fold both ends of the leaf over the filling and, starting with the open side closest to you, roll into a tight cylinder. Repeat with the remaining kale leaves and filling.

 Step 5

Serve with the reserved yogurt sauce.

Tips

Tip: If you have leftover cooked rice, use it for the dolmas. If not, enlist a little help from a precooked rice packet. Watching your sodium? Check the label for added salt.

Nutrition Facts

Serving Size: 4 Stuffed Kale Leaves & 2 Tbsp. Sauce

Per Serving:

471 calories; 16.5 g total fat; 5.6 g saturated fat; 77 mg cholesterol; 748 mg sodium. 607 mg potassium; 48.6 g carbohydrates; 6.4 g fiber; 3 g sugar; 34.5 g protein; 26999 IU vitamin a iu; 228 mg vitamin c; 40 mcg folate; 348 mg calcium; 6 mg iron; 74 mg magnesium;

Exchanges:

4 Vegetable, 3 1/2 Lean Protein, 2 Fat, 1 1/2 Starch

Chickpea Dumplings in Curried Tomato Sauce

Inspired by a dish served in Pakistan, Afghanistan and India called "dharan ji kadhi," our rendition studs the tender chickpea-flour dumplings with chiles and greens. Serve with naan to sop up the sauce for a healthy vegetarian dinner with plenty of protein.

Ingredients

1 cup plus 2 tablespoons garbanzo bean (chickpea) flour (see Tip)

4 cups finely chopped mustard greens or spinach, divided

⅓ cup canola oil plus 2 tablespoons, divided

¼ cup finely chopped red onion

¼ cup whole-milk plain yogurt

¼ cup finely chopped serrano or jalapeño pepper

½ teaspoon salt plus 1/8 teaspoon, divided

2 teaspoons coriander seeds

1 teaspoon cumin seeds

1 teaspoon mustard seeds

1 tablespoon curry powder

1 tablespoon minced fresh ginger

1 (15 ounce) can no-salt-added petite diced tomatoes, undrained

1 (15 ounce) can no-salt-added tomato sauce

Directions

Step 1

Mix flour, 1/2 cup greens, 1/3 cup oil, onion, yogurt, serrano (or jalapeño) and 1/2 teaspoon salt in a large bowl. Using 1 tablespoon to make each, shape into 16 dumplings.

Step 2

Heat the remaining 2 tablespoons oil in a large skillet over medium-high heat. Add coriander, cumin and mustard seeds; cover and cook until they start to pop, about 30 seconds. Stir in curry powder and ginger, then add tomatoes and their juice and tomato sauce; stir to combine. Stir in the remaining 3 1/2 cups greens and 1/8 teaspoon salt. Bring to a simmer.

Step 3

Nestle the dumplings into the sauce, cover and cook, turning the dumplings over and basting with the sauce occasionally, until tender, about 20 minutes.

Tips

Tip: Chickpea flour adds nuttiness and bumps up the nutrition of these dumplings: they boast 2 grams more fiber per serving than dumplings made with all-purpose flour. Look for it with the other specialty flours at well-stocked supermarkets or natural-foods stores.

Nutrition Facts

Serving Size: 4 Dumplings With 3/4 Cup Sauce

Per Serving:

454 calories; 29.2 g total fat; 2.3 g saturated fat; 2 mg cholesterol; 438 mg sodium. 805 mg potassium; 40.6 g carbohydrates; 12.5 g fiber; 13 g sugar; 12.3 g protein; 2424 IU vitamin a iu; 60 mg vitamin c; 11 mcg folate; 190 mg calcium; 4 mg iron; 30 mg magnesium; 1 g added sugar;

Exchanges:

5 1/2 Fat, 3 Vegetable, 1 1/2 Starch